Plant Ba

A Beginners' Guide to Choosing and Adopting a Whole Foods, Plant Based Diet

By Jennifer Marshall

Table of Contents

Introduction

Let's start with a proper introduction.
Hello, my name is Jennifer Marshall. I write books about
health and fitness because I believe that we can always use
more reliable information on it. Having the proper diet is a
hugely important aspect of our ability to thrive in our lives.
I, myself, have seen a lot of people I care about suffer from
poor health and lack of nutritional knowledge. I am fed up
with ignorance being bliss. It is a cop-out. As a writer, I am
always diving deep into the inner workings of life, and
recording what I find. As a health enthusiast, I am always
looking to tweak and improve my own vitality so that I can
better serve our communities. If I have taught you just a
little bit about living a plant based lifestyle, then I did my
job.
I humbly ask you to read through this book with an open
mind and heart. I have included all of the information I
believe you will need to be successful at this. Use your own
intelligence and judgment, and decide what you can use,
and what you will just let fall away; back into the pages of
this book.

Wherever you are on your path, take what I have given you
and let it benefit you however you find it works. Grab a
glass of water maybe a pen and paper, and get comfortable.
I made this book to be a quick read, but a book that is
highly useful for anyone going toward a more plant based
style of diet. I'm here for you if I can be of any benefit, and
I'm honored to get to teach you some things. I will do my
best not to waste your time, because I know it is not in
unlimited supply.
Remember to listen to your body, and your common sense
while reading this book. I will repeat that tip throughout

this book, because it is very important. You know you best. Where you are joined with plant based living is entirely up to you- I am just your guide for now. Thank you for the opportunity.
Here we go…

Chapter 1: What is a Plant Based Diet?

In the most general form, a plant based diet refers to one in which a person eats only foods that are derived from whole, unrefined and unprocessed foods. This is also referred to as a whole food plant based diet. There are many different translations and variations to this diet, but for the most part, it involves avoiding most if not all foods containing animal products, and overly processed food products, a huge emphasis on eating plant based foods that are as close to their natural form as possible. Most plant based eaters stay away from eating meats, dairy, and packaged processed foods. This may be for a number of reasons, and often times the particular foods that are eaten or avoided depend greatly on the reason that person has chosen to adopt the diet.

There has often been some confusion as to whether the plant based diet is just another word for veganism, or if they are a completely different concept with different rules, so let's go into that. There are many similarities between the two, but also some distinct differences. Are veganism and a plant based diet the same thing? The short answer is no. Like I said before, the particular diet that is chosen and the label it is given depends on the individual, and the reason they have chose to live this lifestyle. Many vegans choose to be so because they disagree with the slaughter and poor treatment of farm animals, and so they so not consume these foods. They also usually choose not to use leather, or wear fur or any other animal products. Vegans do not eat any sort of meat, or product containing traces of meat. This includes any broths, or ingredients such as gelatin. Vegans also do not eat any food products that contain ANY ingredient from an animal, including milk or honey. They do not eat any cheese, or yogurt, or margarine or butter, etc. Some slightly more hidden ingredients that contain animal product are whey and casein. These are all avoided. Vegans get most of their food from plant sources, but they are not strictly whole food plant based. They may not be as health conscious, and so many may choose to eat packaged and processed foods, yet stay away from those made of animal. This technically still falls within the parameter of their diet.

Plant based folks eat a primarily plant derived diet- as close to nature as possible. But this does not mean that they are vegan, or even vegetarian. They may simply choose to eat mostly fruits, vegetables, nuts and legumes, etc,. However they may still choose to eat meat, and carefully choose meats that are antibiotics free, grass fed, and lived a free range life. Many plant based dieters believe that meat is still an integral part of a healthy diet, and so they just choose the best quality possible.

Whole food, plant based diets usually take the qualities of both diets, and even go a step further. Keeping foods whole refers to leaving them in their most natural state. So vegetables and fruit are eaten as they are-fresh, frozen or dried without preservatives or added flavor. Nuts are natural, without salt or sugar; grains are not refined or enriched or bleached. Most foods are prepared at home, or in a restaurant where they chefs share the same standards, as to not degrade any of the ingredients or take away any of their nutritional value. Many processed foods use what is known as plant fragments, rather than whole plants. They are reduced, or extracted or otherwise processed in some way.

Whatever the specifics of the diet someone chooses, if they tell you that they are vegan or plant based, you should assume that they do not consume any animal products at all, unless they mention it otherwise. This can help you to avoid accidentally serving them something that they will not be willing or able to eat. And feel free to ask someone about their diet, if you are curious. But make sure that they are willing to talk about it, and also that you listen with an open mind-not looking to judge or challenge their decision to adopt that particular diet.

Now, I would like to clarify the way in which I am using the word diet here. I know that many diets are short term, and involve cutting calories and foods in order to lose unwanted weight. This is a bit of a touchy thing, because there are many diets out there which can put extreme pressure on the body, and will cause weight loss through force or a particular calculation or schedule of eating. This is not what I am referring to in this book. What I will be proposing is that you, the reader, adopt a new addition to your lifestyle that will benefit you, and that you can stick with permanently. This may sound a bit intimidating, to adopt new eating rulcs for life. However, it is my hope that with my help, you will be able to do this painlessly, and really see benefits from it. You may lose weight; you may might have clearer skin and eyes, healthier hair, and even have more abundant energy. And you will help to determine just which benefits you will be rewarded with, by deciding how far you want to go.

The Many Plant Based Diets

In this amazing world of ours there are a million and one ways to get results in something. Everybody is so different, and there are so many of us it's mind-blowing! Everyone has their own opinions and ideas, and tastes. It is no different with food and nutrition. There are many ways to adjust what you eat, when you eat and how much of it you eat. There are plenty of ways to get healthier & a ton of ways to get unhealthy. The type of plant based diet that you choose will depend on your tastes, convictions and ultimate desired results. Such as leather, suede,

Here are a few questions you can ask yourself, to help you narrow down your needs.

1. Will I be eating any meat?
2. Am I eliminating some or all animal products from my diet?
3. If I am eliminating all animal products, will I also choose to eliminate the use of animal products in clothing & around the house, such as leather, suede, and other goods that are made from animal?
4. Are my reasons for switching to this diet due to health, fitness, ethics & morals, medical necessity, or some other reason?
5. What foods am I looking to keep eating?
6. What foods am I looking to add?
7. What are the overall results I am hoping to achieve from this diet?
8. Are there any specific food preferences? Likes? Dislikes?

Now you hopefully have a nice clear picture of your specific needs for this diet. Let's take a look at the most popular, or well-established plant based diets available to follow, whether closely or as a loose translation.

As you see, we already discussed the vegan diets general guidelines in the previous chapter. However, there are also more specific forms of the diet, like the whole foods plant-based diet (which we talk quite a lot about in this book), and the raw vegan diet. The raw diet is basically how it sounds- a vegan diet where none of your food is cooked. More specifically, it is common for raw vegans to eat food that has been cooked, but under a specific temperature; and for a short period of time.

The general temperature for heating food without cooking it and therefore remaining raw is 104 degrees F (40 degrees Celsius), although some argue that the temperature is more like 112F, or even 118F

Another type of vegan is the fruitarian. This variation involves eating all or mostly fruit every day. I personally do not feel that is worth it to eliminate vegetables from the diet because of their huge health benefits. But I have no problem advising you to eat a ton of fresh fruit daily, if you enjoy it! Fruit is so delicious and packed with vitamins and nutrients.

As for vegetarianism goes, there are many options for you to choose from. How far vegetarian do you want to go? If you are not really ready to cut all meat out of your diet, you have the option to go semi-vegetarian. In this case, you would eliminate most meat from your diet. Again, what you choose will be personal to you. I would suggest eliminating all forms of beef and pork from your food, to start. If you want to reduce or omit chicken and other poultry, then that is even better. The decision to eat fish and other seafood or to avoid it is also very important. And of course, there are other types of meat to consider. It will be helpful to think back to what you normally or occasionally eat. Are there any areas of food you are unsure of? Make sure you do your homework, if it is important to you. Including any of these foods, and eliminating certain other types of meat would be considered a semi-vegetarian, or a flexitarian.

For those who choose to exclude all meat from their diet, there are many other levels deeper into vegetarianism.

Lacto-Ovo Vegetarian

The guidelines in the lacto-ovo vegetarian diet state that this type of vegetarian does not eat meat, but may consume dairy products and eggs. This includes all dairy and milk derivatives. Within this diet, honey may be eaten, as well. There is also the option to go organic or free-range with these products.

Ovo-Vegetarian

Ovo-vegetarians practice a vegetarian diet, and have stopped eating or drinking all milk products. However, they still include eggs regularly or once in a while. Ovo-vegetarians may choose to use honey products, or discontinue using them.

Lacto-Vegetarian

With this diet meat and eggs are eliminated, but dairy and milk products are eaten and drank. The choice to eat honey depends on the person in this situation. The reason for including milk will vary, and it may refer to including full-on traditional dairy products, or the hidden milk derivatives that can show up so often in prepared and packaged foods.

Some other, maybe lesser known variations of plant based diets are the macrobiotic diet, and the Mediterranean diet.

The macrobiotic diet focuses a lot on whole food, organic foods, and little to no actual meat. Macrobiotics aims to restore balance by finding the correct relation of yin and yang energies. There is a huge focus on fruits and vegetables and various kinds of whole grains and beans. If you are interested in the macrobiotic diet, I recommend picking up a book from the book store, or from your local library. Of course, you can do some quick research on the internet, as well. Just be sure to check out the source where the article or blog is coming from. Make certain that you are getting your information from a legitimate source. Remember, we want to make the right health decisions because it is so incredibly important to us!

The Mediterranean diet includes light amounts of meats, if at all. It is focused on abundant fruits and vegetables. Also prominent, is the belief that healthy plant based fats are highly beneficial, and should be included often for optimal health.

Chapter 2: Your Why. Motivation to Change

Adopting a new way of life can be many things. It can be intimidating and overwhelming. It can be scary, or feel like the end of having fun eating. It can also be exciting at first, and then prove to be more difficult over time. Sometimes adversity can make you question why you decided to make such a change in the first place. This is why I have decided to create a whole chapter on the subject.

Success in any area requires a significant amount of passion and motivation. You may set up everything else in you environment, to aid in your success, but unless you have the right reasoning why you want it so badly, it will be very difficult to stick with your plan when things get tough.

It is said that 80% of success is having a strong enough WHY (and the right mindset). Only 20% is reliant on mechanics, or what you do. Having a solid motivation is going to be something that you can come back whenever you feel discouraged, or feel frustrated.

You're going to want to choose a motivation that really comes from your heart and passion. Something with a whole lot of powerful emotion behind it. For me, I am a mother, and so my daughter is a <u>huge</u> motivator for me. I want to be my most healthy, so that I can be there for her in every way. Mentally and physically I also want to be a good example, and teach her what foods are the best for our health.

Maybe you have a huge event, or life change that you are preparing for. This can be a great opportunity to get healthier, and into better shape. Some people have an ailment that has been tormenting them for some time. So their reason behind going to a plant based diet may be to experience living pain free, or without the symptoms or side effects.

Whatever your reason for why you want to do this, you should really work toward building it up in your mind. Gain massive leverage for yourself by making a list of everything you will gain by achieving your goals. Make a list of what it will cost you to not make the change. What have you already lost or missed out on, because you haven't changed.

You can even make a list of the possible negativities you may experience by actually changing these aspects of your life. Then you can reexamine these negatives, and see if they are worth keeping things the same over... If not, you can find a solution for them now, before they even become an actual problem.

Now that you have the proper drive (if you don't, go back and work on it until it is solid for you). We will now begin to set small, attainable goals. You will want to be able to track your progress, and know that you are moving in the right direction that you want to go. If you aren't, you want to be able to catch it right away, and correct without too much delay.

With any goal, there are a few things you will want to keep in mind, and there are also a few standard guidelines. First of all, you will want to focus on making SMART goals. This is a pretty common philosophy, and helps achievement happen much quicker. If you are not familiar with the acronym, SMART stands for 5 concepts for achieving goals successfully.

S= Specific

M= Measurable

A= Attainable

R= Relevant/ Realistic

T= Timely/ Time-bound

Specific

You want to paint a clear picture of what your goal is. Know exactly what you want. What is it? What does it look like? Invite all senses, and describe the experience. What is involved?

Measurable

You will have to be able to measure your progress, and keep yourself on the right track. Having a goal that you cannot measure is like going on a trip (especially one that you have never been on), and not having a map. How in the world will you know you are going in the right direction, or if you will ever make it? What is the exact goal, and how will you know when you have arrived there? Find a clear way in which you will measure you goals.

Attainable

In order to really achieve your goals, you must believe deep in your soul that not only are they possible, but also that you yourself can attain them. You also must truly believe that you deserve to achieve this goal. You should shoot high for your dreams, but it is equally important that you actually believe that they are within your reach.

Relevant/ Realistic

There are a couple variations for the 'R' in SMART. Some like to use the word relevant, others prefer to use realistic. Relevant would refer to the bigger picture. Is this goal really important to you and does it fit in with your other goals and overall vision?

Realistic can be used; however, I personally feel that it can tend to reiterate the concepts under the attainable category. Realistic would refer to assuring that your goal is realistically achievable. This seems to be redundant, so I use relevant to reflect on my goals and make sure they are something that I really want in my life. I make sure that it will benefit my life all around, as a whole.

Timely/ Time-bound

There needs to be a specific deadline for each goal that you make. You should know the specific day, month, year that you plan to achieve your goal by. Be sure to make this category realistic as well. Again, aim high, but be sure that it is something you truly believe you can achieve in that particular timeframe. And don't worry too much about miscalculating how much time it will take you. You may need to adjust things according to your circumstances. Sometimes when we are learning something new, we don't realize how long it will actually take, or we may be a bit slower at it, as it is not yet a strong skill of ours. Just begin as best as you can.

The goals you set for adopting the plant based lifestyle will be very personal and relative to you. Depending on your lifestyle, and what you want to achieve, there is a wide range of how you can become more plant based. Some people like to keep their current diet pretty much the same; only adopting a few foods or practices to enhance their health. Some like to change slowly and gradually, until they've completely changed nearly every aspect of their previous diet. Still others may already be well versed in plant based living, and wish to take their commitment even higher; adopting more healthy habits and dropping the disempowering ones.

Go at your own pace. In fact, err on the slower, more gradual side of the scale. Remember, slow and steady wins the race. What kind of race? The one you are running every single day of your life. This is important, and we want it to stick so you can get what you want.

If you're still unsure of what specific goals you want to make, here are some examples:

- Cut out and replace all dairy, by September 17th, this year (*Maybe you'll know you've achieved your goal if you abstained from eating any dairy products for a whole month prior to your deadline, slowly tapering off until cutting it out completely.)

- Lose X amount of excess weight or fat by May 6th, this year. (You may know you've achieved this goal mainly by sticking to a wholesome, nutritious plant based diet.)

- Find X amount of new fruits, vegetables or plant based products that you love eating, and incorporate them into a certain number of meals. (Or learn to cook or prepare it perfectly, say, for a special event).

For each goal you have, go through each category and be sure that you have a powerful reason for attaining it, and keep it somewhere you can easily refer back to during this entire process.

Chapter 3: Benefits and Downsides

Now that you have your own personal reasons for wanting to adopt a healthier diet and lifestyle, you have to power to move forward, and put action to your goals. Here are some of the other reasons that so many people have become plant based eaters. If you had difficulty in the last section, deciding why you personally want this goal, then this chapter will help you to get a better perspective. I have also included some key things to look out for with this diet, and possible downsides. There are undeniably great benefits from adopting a whole food, plant based diet. There are also downsides. As with any lifestyle transformation, there will be a period of adjustment, and also some experiences that may be uncomfortable for you. This book is meant to help make the transition as pleasurable as possible.

Before we go into the benefits, there are a few ideas that I want to make clear. First of all, as powerful as the plant based diet is, it is not the answer to all of your problems, it is not guaranteed to cure all of your ailments and prevent all disease, and I will not bash all other types of diet in favor of this one. This is ultimately about using the best quality of information to decide what is right for your body, and for what you want to achieve. I will do my best to provide enough unbiased information as possible for you, and you will be responsible for forming your own opinions and making your own choices. However, don't be discouraged. Once you figure out how you're going to implement it, this eating style can absolutely help you to make noticeable positive changes in your body, and in your quality of life.

The research results from people who have adopted the plant based lifestyle are pretty astounding. I have poured over page after page of studies and accounts where use of this diet has helped people overcome not just weight issues, but has also helped to clear and prevent numerous diseases and conditions. Most lifestyle-caused ailments can essentially be improved by plant based eating in the very least.

For the most part, a healthy diet is one of the most important things you can do for yourself. We often times forget just the impact that it can have. We are thinking from the outside, almost. We are here-our body's in there; some elusive, scientific world that we don't quite understand. This is why most people just end up going to the doctor for answers, and usually a new type of medication. Unfortunately this will not work if we are seeking true, vibrant health. Pills will only be a cure for some of the symptoms we are experiencing; not for the actual problem. I have been through this myself many times, as well as witnessed it from friends and family. I have had body pains that were only prescribed medicine... Stomach issues? Pills. High blood pressure? Pills. Depression? Pills. As much good as I believe medication is capable, they are not the answer to every single ailment we could have. And many times the side effects can be a whole other issue altogether. Sometimes, they can even be worse than the original problem, which often leads to a switch in your medication to see if results will be better. This guinea pig test can go on for quite some time! You can be left waiting for answers, collecting even more questions.

The solution I want to propose is that we take responsibility for our own bodies, and learn as much as we can about the ways in which they operate. If you are going to be a guinea pig, you may as well be the scientist as well. You will know best how changes feel within yourself. Your doctor should be able to look after areas in which you need to go to medical school to understand. There is a world of knowledge that you can acquire about yourself, that will go a long way toward transforming how you think, feel and look. So let's get discussing the benefits that are available to you, once you adopt the plant based lifestyle.

One of the most sought after benefits of a healthy diet, is of course weight loss. Most people seek a new diet for the promise of losing unwanted fat on their bodies. And although this can seem like a superficial focus, it can be a very good starting off point. It can bring a person to a healthier lifestyle, when they might otherwise never think to look for it Furthermore, losing excess weight can actually do quite a few people a lot of good in their life.

Adopting a whole foods, plant based diet, when paired with a reduction or elimination of animal products, can significantly reduce the amounts of saturated fats, and cholesterol that you consume. This has a dramatic effect on the way your body metabolizes food-especially fats. The fat already in your body gets trapped, because the food we consume usually has so much additional fat that our body must process the incoming foods before getting to our internal food storage. This turns into a cycle, because we are constantly consuming food that our body must find something to do with. The natural, short-term is to place the incoming fat into storage, in case we are ever starving in the future. Unfortunately, this is something that rarely comes in handy for those of us who never seem to be running on empty. The opportunity to use up our stored fat never arises because we just don't give it the chance.

In many cases, those who have adopted this lifestyle, and did it properly were able to lose a significant amount of weight over time. This is mostly because you are eating more vegetables and fruit (very dense in essential nutrients and low in calories), and avoiding foods that are high in calories and very low in nutrients, and disrupt the processes of digestion. Sticking to a whole food, plant based diet (when done properly) can bring about weight loss almost effortlessly. Sounds good to me!

Another one of the benefits of eating this particular diet is that you will be better able to control your insulin and glycemic levels. These two factors have an incredible impact on your health. They affect your hormones, your metabolism, and the levels of hunger that you experience.

One of the deadliest epidemics that we experience in our society is the onset of heart disease and coronary complications. For the most part, the average diet in most developed countries has been high in meats, fat, salt and sugar. These, especially meat, fat and salt, directly affect the performance of the heart and it's joining arteries. The artery walls are the pathways for our blood and oxygen, unfortunately they can be blocked up by plaque- which is caused by cholesterol from animal meat and fat. Once our arteries are blocked enough by plaque, we are in a really bad place. Your blood cannot be properly pumped through your heart, to your brain, and throughout the rest of your body. This is no way to live. The adoption of a plant based diet has been linked very closely with the clearing and strengthening of arterial walls. Real plant based foods can clear the built up plaque, and help to improve blood circulation. It is the only diet ever proven to reverse the #1 killer of men and women (heart disease) in the majority of patients.

One of the main reasons that whole plant based foods work so effectively to lessen bodily diseases and conditions is that most of these foods are highly alkalizing. The modern diet is filled with acidic foods that in turn raise the acidity of the body. This creates an environment in the body that has very little oxygen. An acidic, low oxygen environment is the opposite of what we want in our bodies. This can be a breeding ground for a myriad of harmful bacteria, and death for our healthy bacteria and cells. With this condition, there is usually quite a bit of inflammation, as well. Inflammation is now being tied to nearly every chronic disease there is, from leaky gut syndrome and arthritis, to cancer and heart disease. Anti-inflammatory foods help stop the progression of disease by supplying nutrients that fight oxidative stress (also called free radical damage) including antioxidants, phytonutrients, essential vitamins A, C and E, Trace minerals, electrolytes, and essential fatty acids. **Anti-Inflammatory** foods regulate the immune system, help foster better gut health, boost immune functioning and reduce autoimmune reactions that can cause a cascade of age-related diseases.

Adopting a plant based diet is essentially surrounding yourself with live, nourishing foods. These foods have the building blocks of life that we need to survive, and to grow and thrive. They can be powerful allies against invaders and destruction to your body.

There are a host of devastating diseases (and conditions). Some genetics do play a part in deciding whether a person develops one of them, but it is probably a lot less than you think. Your lifestyle choices play the largest part in your overall health, outside of your access to essential medical care or essential personal care.

The results of a debilitating disease can be such a difficult experience to go through- both for the afflicted as well as their loved ones. I'm sure that in this sort of situation, you are willing to do whatever you can to help ease the pain of those you are close to. Eating whole foods is like giving your body a rescue before it is an emergency. Or maybe it is an emergency, and you need this now more than ever. This is medicinally powerful food that can take your health to the next level. It is no wonder that a plant based diet can have such a huge impact on the state of your body.

So many different diseases can cause harm to our bodies that it can feel like there is always something trying to take us down. Even with our powerful immune systems working in our corner, there are still so many colds, viruses and invaders on the body. Not to mention the chain reaction of inflammation, stress-induced health complications and slow-progressing diseases and chronic conditions we are susceptible to. And unfortunately, most people are completely unaware of how to keep their bodies strong and healthy. They inadvertently set the perfect conditions within themselves for a whole slew of sneaky little health conditions.

This is just a very basic list of some of the diseases and ailments that can be greatly improved by adopting a whole food, plant based diet.

- Alzheimer's; Parkinson's; Dementia
- Cancer; Multiple Sclerosis; Crohn's Disease
- Cataracts; Rheumatoid Arthritis; Ulcerative Colitis
- Diabetes; Gallstones; Kidney Stones
- Diverticulitis; Fibromyalgia; Auto-immune Disease
- Heart Disease; Hypertension; High Cholesterol
- Chronic Acid Reflux; Allergies; Asthma

- Eczema; Acne; Poor Mood
- Premature Aging; Excess Abdominal Fat; Cellulite
- Hormone Imbalance; Metabolic Syndrome; Hypothyroidism
- Chronic Hives; Vaginal Infections; Menstrual Breast Pain in Women
- Headache/ Migraine; Menstrual Cramps in Women; Foul Body Odor
- Oral Health; Cognitive Functions; Gut Health and Flora

Longevity

There is a lot of information and research supporting plant foods' potential to help us live longer. Obviously, if you are putting highly dense nutrients into your body, and keeping disease and illness at bay, then it makes sense that you will be able to naturally live longer (outside of any unexpected freak accidents, of course). So what are the benefits of living longer? Why do we care if we have just a little bit longer of a life? Well, there are so many reasons to strive for longevity. I think that it is a great privilege to be able to share knowledge with those around me for as long as I can. I want to see my daughter grow up to be a mother, or to become what she wants to be. I believe I have a life purpose, to make the world a little bit better because I was alive. The longer I am around, the more I can contribute to the world around me. I think this is a great reason to want to live a longer life.

Plant Based Diets are Better for the Environment

There are other, equally important benefits of having a plant based diet, outside of your health. Producing plant based foods require much less of our natural resources. When compared to factory farming, it is clear that plant farming adds significantly less pollution, CO2, and methane gases into the air. And there is noticeably less demand for precious resources, such as water, soil and fossil fuels.

Here are some fun facts about the costs of production on a typical American factory farm

- More than 9 billion animals are raised and slaughtered each year, for human consumption

- Over 1/3 of all natural materials and fossil fuels are used in animal production in the United States

- Approximately 7 football fields worth of land is leveled every single minute of the day, to create more room for livestock and the food it takes to feed them

- The methane gases emitted by farm animals as they are digesting their food is the same kind of gas that is a contributing factor of the greenhouse effect, which has a massive impact to the state of our environment and is a cause of global warming (a huge imbalance and stress to the quality of our atmosphere

- Natural stretches of land are being bought and turned into farmland all over the world. In the Amazon rainforest, an estimated 70% of land has been turned into farming and grazing land.

- Farms generate over a million tons of manure per day! This is equal to 3 times the amount of that from the entire U.S. population

- Farm animal manure is stored in huge open air lagoons. These massive sources of manure have been known to leak, and have polluted natural water sources. One such spill was recorded to have killed over 110,000 fish.

- Quite often animals are treated with antibiotics in order to protect the meat and accelerate growth or production of the livestock. Excess amounts of antibiotics end up undigested in the animals waste, and in large amounts, as in factory farms, this can contaminate water sources

- It takes approximately 1,581 gallon of water to produce about 1 pound of beef. This is equivalent to the amount for the average American to take 100 showers. It takes only 25 gallons of water to produce 1 pound of whole wheat.

The beautiful thing about our society is that we have the resources, knowledge and technology to make other choices. We have the option to go another route, other than the meat eater lifestyle, if we so choose.

Celebrity Advocates

Celebrities can be a huge influence on our society, and our culture. And we can say that this isn't realistic, of that famous people have extra resources, and it isn't an attainable goal to be able to model what they are doing and eating. You may be partially right. What you see on television and in magazines is only the partial truth of what is actually happening. And sometimes you may see a celebrity drinking a certain meal shake, or eating a certain brand of food, and deem that reason enough to try it for yourself, or try to achieve similar results. There can be a big push for your favorite celebrities to represent products that may not have your best health in mind. It is, again, really important to follow your own instincts, and decide if you are getting your information from a viable source.

However, there are a lot of celebrities out there and just like all humans; there are a lot of them who are good people, who want to do the right thing. There are also some of them that are rotten-let's be honest. But, for the most part, the majority of them are generally good people. And sometimes their influence can lead to so much good in our lives; we never would have known it was possible.

So let's take a look at the celebrities who have chosen to adopt a plant based diet. Perhaps you can relate to some of them, or their ideas behind the switch. Maybe you are already a fan, and you admire them or their work. If you like, you can pick one celebrity and write their name down, or highlight them in this book. You can keep them in mind as a sort or mascot or champion. They can be your inspiration moving forward with the plant based diet.

Alicia Silverstone, *Actress*

Alicia Silverstone has been a strong representative of the plant based lifestyle for many years now. Her life was changed dramatically by the nutritional transformation and she went on to create her own company around her concept of the Kind Diet. This is an animal friendly, vegan diet with which Alicia can share her great love of food blended with

29

her compassion for animals. Alicia has attributed her plant based diet for clearing her acne, helping her to lose unwanted weight, and bringing her a happier existence.

Joaquin Phoenix, *Actor*

Joaquin has had a vegan diet for many years now, after going on a fishing trip, and viewing his experience as a form of inhumane treatment to animals as a boy.

Mayim Bialik, *Neuroscientist/Actress*

Mayim follows a vegan lifestyle not only for animal rights, but for diet and health benefits as well.

Peter Dinklage, *Actor*

The main reason that Peter is a vegan is his amazing compassion for the treatment of animals.

Jared Leto, *Musician/Actor*

"A vegan diet, rich in fruits and vegetables, is full of antioxidants which help protect the body from damage by free radicals."

Jared's diet has been one of the main contributing factors to his seemingly never-ending youthful appearance.

Ellen DeGeneres, *Actress/ Comedian/ TV Personality*

Ellen has chosen a plant based diet to contribute to a cause that she felt was worthy.

Emily Deschanel, *Actress*
Woody Harrelson, *Actor*
Casey Affleck, *Actor*
Natalie Portman, *Actress*
Ellen Page, *Actress*
Lea Michele, *Actress*
Liam Hemsworth, *Actor*
Jessica Chastain, *Actress*
Alec Baldwin, *Actor*
Jenny McCarthy, *Actress*
Michelle Pfeiffer, *Actress*
David Pierce, *Actor*
Tia Mowry, *Actress*
Rooney Mara, *Actress*
Kate Mara, *Actress*
Olivia Wilde, *Actress*
Russell Brand, *Comedian, Actor*
Beyonce, *Musician*

"The benefits of a plant-based diet need to be known. We should spend more time loving ourselves, which means taking better care of ourselves with good nutrition and making healthier choices." —singer Beyonce Knowles

Jason Mraz, *Musician/Activist*

Jason Mraz has made quite an impressive commitment into the plant life. He has commented that he eats mainly raw vegan foods, and that his vegan diet has been a great influence on the music and lyrics he creates. Jason even invested in Café Gratitude, a vegan restaurant in Los Angeles, California.

More Musicians

Sia
Carrie Underwood
Ozzy Osbourne
Stevie Wonder
Miley Cyrus
Bryan Adams
Ellie Goulding
Travis Barker
Ariana Grande
Fiona Apple
Matisyahu
Morrissey
Prince
Thom York

Russell Simmons, *Music Producer*

James Cameron, *Film Director*
"You can't be an environmentalist if you're not eating a plant-based diet. And you can't walk the walk in the world of the future, the world ahead of us, the world of our children, not eating a plant-based diet.
— James Cameron
James Cameron adopted the lifestyle in order to, as he puts it, "save the world". The action director believes in environmentally-conscious practices and sustainability as well.

Thich Nhat Hanh, *Buddhist Monk and Activist*
"Being vegetarian here also means that we do not consume dairy and egg products, because they are

products of the meat industry. If we stop consuming, they will stop producing.

Thich Nhat Hanh chose not to eat meat because he believed in piece between humans and all other species. He felt like eating meat was like inflicting war upon another group of beings.

Kat Von D, *TV Personality/Tattoo Artist*
Steve-O, *Stunt Performer*

Giselle Bundchen, *Model*
 "We all love it. It's not only good for our health and makes us feel good, but it is good for the planet." —model Giselle Bundchen

Pamela Anderson, *Model*
Heather Mills, *Model*
Chris Hedges, *Journalist*
Jim Morris, *Baseball Player*
Pat Neshak, *Baseball Player*

Taj McWilliams-Franklin, *Basketball Player*
"I just wanted to make sure I had a healthy body because I wanted to continue playing for a longer period than most of my peers."

Bill Clinton, *Politician*
Over the years, former President Bill Clinton has gotten some mixed opinions about his decisions. In 2010, though, Mr. Clinton has chosen to make a bold move toward a more plant based lifestyle. He was inspired to do so in order to improve his own health, and well as be a positive example for change. Bill Clinton has talked about vegetarianism and veganism as a promising

solution for our nation's poor health epidemic. Bill says that the plant based diet makes him "feel good."

"It changed my whole metabolism and I lost 24 pounds and I got back to basically what I weighed in high school." — President Bill Clinton
Al Gore, *Politician*

David Carter, *Football Player*

 Carl Lewis, *Olympic Athlete*

Steph Davis, *Professional Rock Climber*
"I started eating vegan because I noticed that it made me feel better and perform better. After a couple of years, I became aware of factory farming, and what exactly is being done to animals all day every day in our society in order to create cheap meat, eggs and dairy products that are not even causing Americans to be healthy or fit. Knowing what I know now, even if being vegan didn't make me healthier, energetic and stronger (which it does); I would continue to eat this way purely in order to keep my dollars out of the system that perpetuates cruelty and abuse."

Mike Tyson, *Boxer*

Nate Diaz, *MMA Fighter*

Luke Cummo, *MMA Fighter*

 Many more celebrities and influential people follow a plant based diet; you would be amazed!! You might find, if you do a little research of your own, you will be able to find a plant-loving warrior who really inspires you!

Some Words of Caution

When it comes to this lifestyle, there are numerous reasons why it is beneficial and can have tremendous positive effects. But like anything, your plant based diet will not be perfect. And there will be a substantial period of adjustment. You may notice that some foods may not sit well with you. There is also the possibility that you don't presently eat quite enough fiber in your diet. Switching to a high-fiber diet can sometimes cause some stomach discomfort, or gas. This will lesson as your body has adjusts to the amount of healthy enzymes to break down your food better-even those tough bits of hearty fiber. I wouldn't really say that this lifestyle has any actual downsides to it, but I will say that there may be some adjustments, while you are getting the hang of things. Here are the most common complaints, and tips on how to ease or eliminate them.

Deficiencies

The main deficiency you need to be aware of is a lack of Vitamin D. Our bodies do not produce Vitamin D naturally, so we must get it from either our food, or an over-the-counter vitamin. I wouldn't let this deficiency deter you from a plant based diet at all, however. Actually, most people are deficient in vitamin D. Most people are not making sure that they get enough of it. The reason why it is particularly important for vegans and vegetarians is that it is not available in plant based foods. It comes from animal meat. This is an easy fix, though, with a simple multivitamin with B12, or a B12 complex on its own. A little bit of sunshine helps a lot, too!

Discomfort

Let's face it; indigestion is not a pretty picture. But it can be a fact of life, if your body is not prepared to take on the food you are eating. If you are used to a relatively low-fiber diet, with not as many plants as the as the plants based diet has, you may not have the natural enzymes in your gut needed to process high-fiber foods. Most beans and legumes require a particular enzyme to break down and be digested. The problem is that our bodies do not make this enzyme. But don't worry! This is a temporary discomfort for the greater good. Besides, there are ways to ease this problem, and often times eliminate it.

Tips to ease to transition:
- Stay hydrated; drink as much water as possible! This will help to flush out your body, and keep everything moving along easier.

- Incorporate high fiber foods into your diet very gradually. This can especially be true with rougher fibers, like broccoli; and also with beans and legumes. With lentils, start out by eating only about 2 tablespoons per day, and gradually building up to a quarter cup, a half of a cup, and so on.

- Soak your dry beans for 1-3 days prior to cooking- the longer the better. This will break down those tricky enzymes. Soak them in very warm water, alkaline or at least filtered. Drain the water, and replace with very warm water 3 times per day, to rinse away any residuals.

- Cook beans low and slow- all day if possible.

- Some say that cooking your beans and legumes in a broth will help to reduce the discomfort they provide, but there is no known reason why this works.
- Serve your beans and lentils with fermented foods, to aid digestion
- Place a strip of kombu (sea vegetable) in the water with your beans and legumes. Kombu contains the enzyme that breaks down their rougher fibers.

Chapter 4: THE FOOD

Now let's get down to the real business at hand. What do we get to eat, and what are we eliminating? It is best to have this decided, but you can always make changes as you become more accustomed. Everybody has different tastes and dislikes, so the more thought you put into this area, the more clear your guidelines will be.

In order to get the best out of your plant based diet, you will want to set a path and boundaries for yourself. This will help to ensure your success, and help you to maximize your results. The best way to go about this is to make it as fun and enjoyable for you as possible! Make yourself templates and sample lists and menus that will inspire you, and help you decide what will work best for you. Start out with a pen or pencil, and paper. Write down what you currently eat. Try to get the clearest idea of what you eat day in and day out. You may want to keep a food journal for about a week, but for some this won't be a pleasurable experience. But what you can do is think of all of the foods that you normally eat, be entirely honest, and place them each in one of two categories: Do Eat, and Do Not Eat.

The foods you will continue to eat, you will place under Do Eat. The foods you will plan to avoid, at least temporarily, you will place under Do Not Eat. Seems simple enough, right? Now, you should do this slowly, and over time. Choose only a few foods to adopt, and to eliminate from your diet at a time. This will be a gradual transition. You may even want to make a third category marked Why? This category is a great place to note why you are choosing to add or eliminate that food, in case you need a reminder.

Here are some examples of **foods to add** (Do Eat, or whatever you decide to name it)

Vegetables

Kale

Broccoli

Cucumber

Celery

Ginger

Sweet Potato

Bell Peppers

Carrots

Corn

Cucumbers

Garlic

Ginger

Mushrooms

Onions

Potatoes

Tomatoes (technically fruit)

Avocado (also a fruit)

Zucchini

Fruit

Banana

Apple

Orange

Grapefruit

Grapes

Pineapple

Berries

Lemons and Limes

Pears

Grains

Brown Rice

Sprouted or Gluten Free Bread

Rice or gluten free Noodles

Quinoia

Steel Cut Oats

Tortillas or Taco shells

Proteins

Tofu

Tempeh

Beans

Lintels

Nuts

Nut Butters

Seeds

Chia Seeds

Chickpeas

Edamame

Flax Seed

Hummus

Quinoia

Tahini

(Dark Leafy Green Vegetables)

Pantry Essentials

Frozen Foods

Dairy-free ice cream/ sorbets

Frozen Veggies

Frozen Fruit

Condiments

Hot Sauce

Ketchup

Tahini

Soy Sauce

Canned Goods

Beans

Coconut Milk

Tomatoes

Tomato Paste

Bouillon Cubes

Dried Fruit

Nutritional Yeast

Oils

Olives

Marinara Sauce

Vinegars

Agave Syrup

Vanilla Extract

Baking Soda

Baking Powder

Chocolate, dark or dairy free

Cocoa powder, unsweetened

Sugar

Flour

Maple Syrup

Spices

Basil

Black Pepper

Chili Powder

Ground Cinnamon

Ground Cumin

Curry Powder

Garam Masala

Garlic Powder

Onion Powder

Oregano

Paprika

Rosemary

Salt (iodized)

Ground Turmeric

Thyme

Foods to Eliminate

Adding the right life-supporting foods to your life will go a long way toward helping you achieve the health you desire.

40

It will give you the nutrients and enzymes to make your body work harmoniously. However adding helpful foods is only part of the food equation. Your body is constantly working to build healthy cells, and to discard of the dead unhealthy material. This process of detoxification is an essential body function. It protects us against destructive toxins and damaged cells. Left unchecked without being removed these toxins can wreak havoc on your, and has the potential to destroy perfectly healthy cells and organs. The detoxification process is just as important as eating nutrient rich foods. The absolute best way to remove unhealthy foods and harmful toxins from your body is to avoid eating them in the first place.

I have composed a basic list of foods and ingredients that should be removed from your kitchen, and your everyday diet. Eliminating these foods will help you achieve the cleanest possible dietary health.

Reduce or Eliminate:

All animal products

Honey (if going full vegan, or eliminating for any reason)

Dairy products

High fructose corn syrup (All refined sugars)

Partially hydrogenated oils

Enriched/ bleached flours

Foods with a very long list of unnatural ingredients

Monosodium glutamate

Foods enriched or fortified with unnatural vitamins

*This happens when the food has been extracted, and separated from its natural state. It is then usually added with essential trace elements and vitamins. This is not the way we want to consume our food.

Side note: Usually the fact that foods that have long scientific sounding ingredients means that they were made in a lab. This doesn't fair well once in the body.

Learning to Read Labels

Adopting a new eating style and becoming more aware of what is coming into your body can be a pretty overwhelming endeavor. But with the right knowledge and a lot of practice, you will be able to find out what is in anything you are eating, and you will be able to decide for yourself if it is something that you will choose to eat. The first step to improving something is awareness. Once you have a better idea of what goes into your food, you can move away from the unnatural foods and closer to natural, wholesome nutrition.

Nutrition Facts

Serving Size 1 oz (28g)
Serving Per Container 2

Amount Per Serving

Calories 100	Calories from Fat 15

	% Daily Values*
Total Fat 1.5g	**2%**
Saturated Fat 0.5g	**3%**
Trans Fat 0g	
Cholesterol 35mg	**12%**
Sodium 580mg	**24%**
Total Carbohydrate 1g	**0%**
Dietary Fiber 0g	**0%**
Sugars 1g	
Protein 21g	**42%**

Calcium 2%	•	Iron 8%

* Percent Daily Values are based on a 2,000 calorie diet. Your Daily Values may be higher or lower depending on your calorie needs.

	Calories	2,000	2,500
Total Fat	Less than	65g	80g
Sat Fat	Less than	20g	25g
Cholesterol	Less than	300mg	300mg
Sodium	Less than	2400mg	2400mg
Total Carbohydrate		300g	375g
Dietary Fiber		25g	30g

Here I have included a brief lesson on deciphering your nutritional facts.

For many people, the nutritional facts on a food means very little, when it comes to making food choices. For one, it can be a challenge to understand exactly how nutritional information correlates to what is going on in your body. I think that the number or calories is probably at the most basic level understanding how to use food labels. Basically, you need a certain amount of calories per day, to maintain your body weight and current level of nutrition. Your body uses a certain range of calories daily, just by being alive and moving around. The more physical activity you get, the more calories are burned. The more calorie-filled foods you eat, the more calories are stored in your body, usually as fat. Having more muscle on your body means that you can burn more fat.

There are, of course, many other factors that come into play when your body metabolizes food.

Macros & Vitamins

Another basic gauge for judging your food's nutritional value is the division or macros. What is your meal primarily composed of? This is referring to the type of food, and how it will generally be used in the body. Fat, protein and carbohydrates make up your macros. Also important are the amount of sugar and the amount of salt.

Fat

Fat is either used immediately in the presence of physical activity, or it will be stored as fat in the body. Fat is stored up in case we are ever faced with a food shortage and need to be protected against starvation. In most developed countries, unless you have a specific life complication where you go hungry often, we do not have a food storage. We have a surplus of calorie-dense food that is devoid of any nutrition. This is where much of our excess fat comes from.

But all fats are not created equal. Our bodies actually really need fat to be healthy, lustrous, and to feel satisfied by our meals. You want to get plenty of good fats in your diet to keep the right balance. Healthy fats are unrefined, and come mostly from plants, nuts and seeds. Truth be told, healthy fats can also be found in certain types of fish and seafood. Things like avocados and coconut oil provide wonderful healthy fats. So do nuts and seeds like flax and chia. Snack on plenty of nuts and seeds!

Protein:

This nutrient is the main ingredient to building our cells and muscles. Protein is what gives us our lean, powerful muscles. Protein helps us to metabolize fat, and helps to regulate your blood sugar. It also benefits your physical performance abilities, not to mention it also really helps to fill you up without having to eat a lot of extra calories. With the right combination, you can make protein work for you to create the body and the health you strive for.

Carbohydrates

This is essentially your sugar, for your physical energy. Your carbohydrates are either filled with a good source of fiber, or turned into sugar- to be used immediately, or stored as fat.

When it comes to the ingredients list, the first 5 ingredients make up most of that food, and contain about 95% of the whole. All ingredients descend in order of concentration. Look out for chemical-laden ingredients which are hard to pronounce, and sound unfamiliar or not descriptive of what it is originally derived from. Look for whole ingredients that are un-tampered with. And if you choose to eat something you know has unhealthy ingredients, then make sure you enjoy it, count it as a treat (or cheat meal), and make up for it moving forward at the next meal.

I also want you to be aware of the order in which your food is digested. Different foods have different schedules of when they enter and exit the body. They also require different enzymes and ph balances to be properly digested. Now, if you have quite a strong gut, you may not need this step. But if you are experiencing noticeable digestive issues, then food combining may make a big difference for you.

Here is a general guideline for combining your foods effectively and each foods approximate digestion time

Eat melon alone (takes 15-30 minutes)

Eat fruits alone (1-2 hours)

Starches like grains, roots, beans, and bread items can be eaten with vegetables (3 hours)

Proteins like nuts, seeds beans and meat go great with vegetables (4 hours, but animal protein can take 8 hours or longer)

Avoid mixing protein and starched. They do not work well together.

Avoid mixing fruit and protein- or starch and fruit. This can create rotting in the gut.

Enjoy avocados with just about anything!

Veggies are compatible with anything!

Special Diets & Substitutions

If you have a specific food allergy, you know the importance scanning your food ingredients, and assuring it isn't there. One of the great things about the plant based diet is that you can adapt it, and you don't have to stick to a specific set of meals to get the positive results. You can make substitutions, or a different recipe altogether, if you can't find a way around that particular ingredient.

Common Food Allergies

Peanuts

Tree nuts

Milk

Eggs

Fish

Shellfish

Coconut Oil (some auto-immune diseases)

Gluten, Wheat or Certain Grains (Celiac Disease)

Chapter 5: How to Get Started

This chapter will teach you how to put everything into action.

In order to get started on the right foot, you'll need to get into the right headspace for the changes you are incorporating into your life. Having the right mindset for change and for your health will go a long way to help you to be effective and successful at this.

It is amazing just trying to imagine the amount of power your mental state and thoughts can have on your life, and on your decisions. How do we assure that your mind is working on your side? By guiding your opinions and perceptions. And by trying consciously to maintain a positive attitude. Just an overall willingness to do what it will take. You must find, and hold, the strength to commit to new habits; replacing old ones. You are making a commitment to tread into territory that is mysterious to you. You need to be open to fail a little, and try something new.

The plant based diet can have a lot of different connotations along with it. Sometimes having a strong misconception can be a roadblock, if you let it color your beliefs and choices. Try to keep an open mind going into this change. Many people have the perception that, for example, vegan food is tasteless. Or that this type of eating has to be difficult. You may agree, or think that it is impossible to get the proper nutrients on a plant based diet. Many people also believe that eating this way must be super expensive. You will find your own path and beliefs as you learn to experiment more. I will give you all of the tools that I can, but you have to be willing to explore and experiment to find your path.

There are many ways to go about change, and what you choose will be based on a variety of things. Some people prefer to transition very slowly in order to make the adjustment not such a shock, and also to pay more attention to the process over long term. Others like to completely change their life over the course of a month, week or even overnight. Some people have a lot of fears revolving around change, and some people may have a sense of urgency around the subject, because of a certain upcoming event with a specific date.

The method I prefer, and the one I will discuss in this book, is the steady, gradual change that has a clear direction and purpose. I find that this is the best way to build solid habits, and a stronger foundation under your new construction of healthy habits. Let's get down to it!

Stocking the Kitchen

I want you to think of your kitchen as your strongest ally on the road to greater health. Are you inspired? Feel free to switch up the décor in your kitchen to make it more meaningful, and to make it more conducive to preparing and eating healthy meals. You want to feel inspired, and in control of yourself when you walk in the kitchen to create a meal or grab a snack. If you find that you don't have everything that you need to have the experience, you can plan to slowly gather acquire these items over time; and improvise the rest. While you are making the transition to vegetable proteins, be sure to check out the many types of mock meats, or textured vegetable proteins available. Yes, some may be overly processes, but it can definitely be a great alternative to animal meats. This can be especially helpful when you are just starting to make the transition. Once you are accustomed to not eating meat, or eating very little, you can start to move away from the more processed versions and move toward more wholesome options.

I will give you a glance at what I recommend stock the house with in order to get the best results and to enjoy some pretty delicious food!

What to keep in the kitchen

It may be tempting to just go into your kitchen and toss everything out, starting from scratch. More than likely, though, you still have some foods that are worth keeping around. Take a look in there, and acknowledge the foods you have that are beneficial for you. Everything else can go. It may be more enjoyable to enlist a helper for this job, or you may want to tackle it all yourself like a nutritional warrior. Either way, we are going to separate the good from the ugly. I like to start in the pantry and cupboards, pull every single item out, put it on the table or counter and begin sorting objectively. You can separate the food you are eliminating into 3 categories- toss; pass on and donate. You can pass any items on that you thing a friend or family member will use (this can also be nice for when an item is open, but still good. Any unclaimed food that is still in good condition can be donated to a local shelter or food closet.

Kitchen appliances and tools

Blender

Good Pan

Cutting boards

Mixing bowls

Good knife

Food storage containers

Baking Sheet

Colander

Spiralizer

Vegetable peeler

Can opener

Garlic press

Mandolin slicer

Juicer

Citrus Juicer

Meal Planning

For this next step, it may be beneficial for you to first spend some time recording what you normally eat day to day. I would do this for two weeks, while tracking calories as well. This will give you a good idea of the type of foods you typically eat. You can find your average daily calories and decide what adjustments need to be made.

Leave an allowance of one page for each day, and write down everything you ate (time would be helpful here too, but don't worry if you're not quite ready for that yet). Also include what meals you ate them for and the calories (if you are tracking calories). Remember: Make sure to record EVERYTHING that you eat. This is important.

Next take that information and analyze it. What are your go-to foods? Are you eating calories way beyond your needs? Way less? Do you tend to lean toward sweets & sugary foods? Or how about spicy or salty? If you are recording times of your meals, ask yourself how often you get hungry. Note the size of your meals, how often you get hungry, when you are at your hungriest, and when you crave to snack.

Once you have recorded in your food journal for two weeks, and you have gathered the information you need, you can make the necessary adjustments. What food did you eat, that you will be eliminating from your diet. Are there any go-to foods that you need to substitute for something healthier? Are there any flavors that you love, but need a better version for? You really can collect so much information from this little bit of data collecting.

Now we will work on building menu plans for you.

If you are still wanting to track your calories, and assuming you are eating 3 meals and 2 snacks per day, you will take your target daily calories and divide it by 4. This will give you the value of each of your 3 meals. Next divide that number by 2, and you have the value for each of your snacks. Now this will be a general guideline for how many calories should be in each meal and snack.

So for example, say you are eating 1,200 calories a day (this is only an example. Keep in mind that this is the minimum amount of calories an adult should have daily, and it is recommended for those of us who are around 5', like me).

You would divide that number by 4, which is 300. So each meal would be 300 calories. Divide that number by 2, and you get 150. So each snack would be 150 calories.

Use this guideline during the meal planning process. You can decide whether you like to meal plan better on paper, or on a computer word document. I like to do a little bit of both. Also, experiment with formats to find what suits you. For each day of the week, leave a space for breakfast, lunch, and dinner with 2 snacks (also the occasional dessert!). It is also helpful to plan out your beverages, if you are looking to improve that as well. But you can allow yourself unlimited pure water and unsweetened tea. Keep in mind, black tea is much more acidic. I tend to stick with variations of green tea.

As an extra tip, I find it really helps to repeat as many of my meals day-to-day, as possible, while still enjoying those meals. It can really work to reduce the amount of time and effort planning and prepping them. Also tracking their calories will be easier.

Planning Meals & Writing the Shopping List

Create a word document or grab a pen and some paper, and make a quick shopping list of what you need. What groceries are running low? Next brainstorm meals that you want to have for the week. Take a glance through local store deals, coupons, and sales.

You may find it easier to build your menu plan starting with you dinners. This can sometimes be beneficial, especially when you tend to have dinner with family, friends, colleagues or your significant other. If this isn't your family dynamic, no worries! You can choose what meals you would like to start with, and fill in the other meals and snacks until you have a plan for all of your meals for the week. Just being this prepared can make life so much easier, and assure you will be prepared to make healthier food choices.

Find out what you need to buy for your meals and add them to your grocery list.

Here is a sample menu plan for the week, and a companion grocery list:

Monday

 Breakfast: Oatmeal; Fruit

Lunch: Vegan Chili; bread

Dinner: Veggie teriyaki with rice

Snacks: Fruit; Granola; Nuts

Tuesday

Breakfast: Tofu scramble; Veggies

Lunch: Burrito Bowl

Dinner: Lentil Stew

Snacks: Fruit; Trail Mix; Veggies and Hummus

Wednesday

Breakfast: Oatmeal; Fruit

Lunch: Veggie Sushi Rolls

Dinner: Tacos; Beans and Rice

Snacks: Fruit; Dark Chocolate; Seeds

Thursday

Breakfast: Smoothie Bowl

Lunch: Veggie Wrap

Dinner: Veggie Burgers and Homemade French Fries

Snacks: Fruit; Dried Veggies; Veggie and Hummus

Friday

Breakfast: Tofu Scramble, veggies

Lunch: Sprouted Grain Veggie Sandwich

Dinner: Veggie Teriyaki with Tofu

Snacks: Fruit; Trail Mix; Granola

Saturday

Breakfast: Breakfast Wrap

Lunch: Veggie Wrap

Dinner: Lentil Stew

Snacks: Fruit; Veggies and Dip; Wine

Sunday

Breakfast: Green Smoothie

Lunch: Sprouted Grain Sandwich

Dinner: Veggie Burgers with Homemade French Fries

Snacks: Fruit; Granola; A Special Dessert Item for once a week

Making Your Grocery List

Fruit:

Apples

Bananas

Cucumber

Pineapple

Watermelon

Lemon or Lime

Vegetables

Lettuce

Tomatoes

Onions

Carrots

Celery

Cucumbers

Avocados

Broccoli

Cauliflower

Potatoes

Garlic

Spinach

Refrigerated/ Dairy or Alternatives:

Soymilk/ milk

Margarine

Hummus (or you can make your own)

Tofu

Canned Goods:

Pineapple

Refried Beans

Garbanzo Beans

Tomatoes

Tomato paste

Dry Goods:

Rice

Nori Sheets (for sushi)

Oatmeal

Sea Salt

Dark Chocolate

Spices

Granola

Nuts

Seeds

Dried Veggies

Spices

Lentils

Beans

Bread/ Cereal:

Oatmeal

Pita Bread

Wrap or tortilla

Sprouted Grain Bread

Frozen Foods:

Edamame

Spinach

Strawberries

Etc:

Vegan Mayonnaise (or use hummus)

Ketchup

Hot Sauce

Soy sauce

Hoisin Sauce

Honey

Optional:

Wine

Special Dessert

Chapter 6: Money Saving Tips

One of the reasons some people give for not eating healthy, whole ingredient foods, is that they believe it will be too expensive to maintain. And it can be true to a certain extent. It can be tricky to find good-quality organic produce for a low cost. And sometimes they less expensive stores do not have the best selection of quality fruits and vegetables. I have experienced this for myself, and have found ways to get the most for my money. First of all, I remember where I can get the best deal each item. You can make a note of this, or start a word document to help you keep track of your money saving strategies. I like to buy some of my heartier, less fussy produce at a more inexpensive store, and go to the more higher-end health food-friendly stores for my more finicky foods-like berries, and peaches. Shopping around at too many different stores can make things more complicated, but picking a few stores that tend to compete may be in your best interest.

There are many ways that you can save money while still eating wholesome foods. Some of them may work perfectly well for you, and others you can discard.

One of the best ways to avoid extra costs is to plan your meals ahead of time. This will give you a better sense of control and preparation for the week ahead, which will cut down on extra trips to the store. You can plan a certain day of the week to batch your grocery store trips.

Another highly effective way to reduce unnecessary and unhealthy purchases is to make sure that you are not hungry when you go food shopping. Actually, I don't recommend doing any kind of shopping hungry-it's just not pleasant. I know eating before grocery shopping is not a new suggestion, but it is worth repeating. It works. Every time I go to the grocery store hungry, I end up with more snacks and sweet treats in my cart, on top of the meal I plan to eat when I get home; most of the time they are foods that I wouldn't have picked up, had I eaten a proper meal beforehand. So if possible, eat at least a little something before you take on the grocery store.

It can be in your benefit to scan through the sales of your local stores, to see if there is some extra money to save on the groceries you already plan to buy. This is key- seeing items being on sale (even a really great sale) do not mean that you should buy foods that you don't need and weren't already buying. Some stores provide a club with loyalty rewards. You can take advantage of these and plan your shopping list around it. For items that aren't on sale, you can sometimes find coupons that can really help lower your overall cost. (Again, only use coupons for items you are planning to buy already. Unnecessary costs, even if at a discount, still cost you extra money.) Store apps may be worth looking into, as well. They can notify you when there is a sale, or certain foods that have been discounted.

Sometimes you can find better deals for the amount of food you get, if you shop at your local farmers markets; and ethnic food stores as well. Get to know them and see if they will work in your shopping routine.

Another good strategy is to buy your dry goods in bulk. You can really buy any foods that you are sure to eat before they go bad. Dry goods just tend to stay fresh longer (nonperishable).

Also, buying your foods when they are in season serves more than one purpose. You can save money on produce that is more readily available, and you can also benefit from getting the best tasting food because it is at its peak state of freshness.

Decide if any of these tips resonate with you, and help make your life easier. You really can save a surprising amount of money, when you put enough focused attention on it.

Chapter 7: The Way to Persevere

This chapter goes hand in hand with your driving force to achieve your goals. Persevering requires continuing on your intended path, even after it has been a while and it may not be easy. Sometimes a goal or change can be so clear and compelling that there is no question whether you can achieve it. However, after a period of time the reasons behind your motivation may be forgotten or may not have the same power they had before.

The key is to revive that original force. Make it as fresh as it was when you first made it. There are many ways to do this, and we will discuss some of them in this chapter. Keep an open mind as you read the tips I've provided, and see if any of them will work for you and your goals.

Sometimes it can take just one idea to set a spark; or to rekindle one. One great idea has the potential to push you through even the most difficult struggles. It can take you all the way through those struggles, towards your greatest achievements. And any obstacles you make it through builds your strength and determination. Losing your motivation can be a tragedy, when you know you have so much potential and unachieved goals. And sometimes you may even lose the progress you were building before you lost track. This can be such a shame. I have seen it happen to other people, and I have experienced it for myself. My goal is to prevent this for myself and to help others avoid it as well.

The first thing that I like to do when I lose motivation, for something I am working on, is to find that place where I was originally inspired. What made me create that goal or commitment in the first place? Was it something I saw or read? Did I speak with someone about it? Was it a thought I had, or state I was in? I find that I can at least spark my interest again if I take the right actions to remind myself. Just a little inspiration can go a long way toward retrieving your driving force.

Re-examine all of the work you did in chapter 2, in which we built up your WHY power. What are your reasons for wanting to achieve your goal? Are your reasons still valid for you? If not, discover some new reasons you want to achieve your goals. In thing case, why you want to improve your health, and adopt a plant based diet.

Another great way to rebuild your motivation is to see how far you have come. Look back to where you first started making changes. Have you made a lot of improvements? If so, be sure to applaud yourself for your progress. This will help you to see the value in doing what still needs to be accomplished.

Chapter 8: FAQ

Here are some of the most asked questions regarding the plant based diet. Hopefully this section will help to answer any questions that weren't answered for you in the rest of the main section of the book.

Which is better for you-a vegan or a vegetarian diet?

The answer to this really depends on your lifestyle and what you are trying to achieve. Also, you need to be aware of what you are willing to commit to. I personally do not eat dairy (due to an allergy), so not eating dairy is easier for me. So veganism is my diet of choice, but what you choose must be your own personal decision. Make it wisely!

Is yeast vegan?

Technically, mushrooms and yeast aren't "plants" since they belong to the Fungi kingdom, but these foods are eaten by vegans and people who follow a "plant-based diet". They are often included in the plant category- as are mushrooms.

Can you eat bread as a vegan?

Traditionally bread is made from yeast, flour and water, and so yes it is suitable for vegans, most of the time. Some commercially sold breads contain dairy or eggs so be sure to check ingredients before you purchase.

What is a minimally processed plant based food?

Minimally processed foods are tampered with only to a certain extent. This is mostly important because these kinds of foods can still maintain their nutritional value. Guacamole is an example of a plant food that is minimally processed or prepared.

Hummus, applesauce, salsa, peanut butter, oatmeal, and vegetable broth would be other examples.

Condiments such as mustard, hot sauce, vinegars, and soy sauce are also generally accepted as within the scope of "minimally processed".

Corn tortillas, whole-grain breads (e.g. whole-wheat bread), and pastas

How do vegans get enough protein?

There is really no need to worry about becoming deficient in protein if you are consuming enough calories to live. Humans cannot actually be deficient in protein unless they are starving. You can get all of the complete protein you need from plant sources.

Is it healthy for children to be on a vegan diet?

Yes, a vegan or vegetarian diet is a healthy part of an infant or child's life, as long as enough attention is paid to balance and wholesome plant based foods in the right amounts, but this is true with any regular diet.

How do I get enough calcium on a vegan diet? What about osteoporosis?

You will get plenty enough calcium with this eating, because you will be eating a lot of dark leafy greens, like broccoli and spinach; and from other plant sources like white beans, soy, almonds and rice. Also, you will get high amounts of all other life-building nutrients, as well. Exercise will also contribute to your prevention of osteoporosis.

Avoid calcium destroyers like tobacco, caffeine and excess salt.

What's wrong with drinking milk? Is organic milk better? Is soymilk a safer alternative? What about other dairy products?
Cow's milk is not the worst thing for you on the planet; but it is a rich source of cholesterol, saturated fat, and possibly added chemicals and hormones unless clearly stated.

Is it safe to eat soybeans and other soy foods?
Soy beans in their natural state are perfectly safe and healthy for you. Once you get into the more processed and packaged soy products, you run the risk of eating not-so-healthy vegetarian foods. Tofu should be fine, and is recommended. Edamame is an awesome protein-packed snack. And soymilk is processed to an extent, but a vast improvement from traditional cows' milk.

Are carbohydrates bad for you? Is it OK to eat carbohydrates if I am trying to lose weight?
Carbohydrates should not be labeled as an enemy, or as something you need to avoid, if you want to lose weight. Much of the country would probably want to lose weight if they knew they could. The key is to focus on whole plant based starches, and healthy grains. Whole grains, potatoes, whole wheat pasta, brown rice, and sweet potatoes. Avoid

processed versions, which have lost much of their fiber and other nutrients.

Should I be on a gluten-free diet?
If you are experiencing any of the possible side effects of gluten intolerance, then a gluten-free diet would be beneficial to you. If you would like to see if eliminating gluten from your diet would make a positive difference in your health, then I would highly recommend it! You can try it out as a temporary experiment, and see how your body responds. Remember to always listen for your body's signals. There is a lot we don't know, that our body can tell us. Listen and learn.

Doesn't a vegetarian or vegan diet require a lot of planning and preparation?
Your diet is as easy of complicated as you want it to be. But I will say, and I believe many would agree with me, that proper planning and reparation will work beautifully in your favor in life. This is covered more in the section I have on meal planning.

CAN YOU GET FULL EATING ONLY PLANTS?
Yes, of course! Plants have a ton of fiber and protein, which fill you up the most. And they also provide you with the majority of your vital nutrients and vitamins. These foods will keep you fuller for longer; with less water retention and bloating as in traditional animal-based dishes.

Conclusion

I would like to thank you from the bottom of my heart, for reading my book. I really do appreciate it. The reason why I wanted to write this book is because I feel that there is a need for more quality information; that is available to anyone. I wanted to take all of the knowledge that I have learned about plant based diets, and share it where it is needed. Having the right information is key if you want to make the most informed decisions in your life. Unfortunately, in the health and diet industry there is plenty of misleading information, and it can be confusing and frustrating. Don't go for the quick fix. Stick to the most sustainable, logical, healthy habits. It is said that it takes somewhere between 3 weeks and one month to create a habit. So stick with it, and I am sure you will experience so many health benefits; you will be amazed at what you can accomplish. It is my deepest hopes that this book has been helpful to you. I hope that I have helped to bring you closer to the health you want to gain for yourself.

I would love to hear from you! Please feel free to send me an email with any questions. I am always glad to help you further improve your health and your nutritional diet.

You can contact me at:

Cleverdaydream@gmail.com

Resources

https://www.mindbodygreen.com/0-952/PlantBased-Diet-for-Beginners-How-to-Get-Started.html

https://happyherbivore.com/2013/07/what-is-plant-based-diet-difference-from-vegan/

http://yumuniverse.com/how-to-start-a-plant-based-diet/

http://www.zliving.com/food/food-drink/what-is-whole-food-plant-based-diet-see-the-guide

http://myplantbasedfamily.com/getting-started/

https://en.wikipedia.org/wiki/Plant-based_diet

http://health.usnews.com/best-diet/best-plant-based-diets

http://www.onegreenplanet.org/natural-health/whole-foods-plant-based-fifty-dollars-a-week/

https://www.reddit.com/r/PlantBasedDiet/

https://nutritionfacts.org/topics/plant-based-diets/

http://www.huffingtonpost.com/entry/plant-based-diet-vs-vegan-diet_us_5923374fe4b034684b0ebff0

https://draxe.com/plant-based-diet/

https://www.plantbasedcooking.com/recipes/

"The China Study" by Dr. T. Colin Campbell

https://www.farmsanctuary.org/learn/factory-farming/factory-farming-and-the-environment/

http://www.onegreenplanet.org/animalsandnature/facts-on-animal-farming-and-the-environment/

http://www.self.com/story/vegan-diet-pros-cons

Leave a review!

Finally, if you enjoyed this book, then I'd like to ask you for a favor, would you be kind enough to leave a review for this book on Amazon? It helps me out a lot, and it'd be greatly appreciated!

Visit this book's page on Amazon to leave a review

https://www.amazon.com/dp/B074SGK7K1

Thank you and good luck!

Check Out My Other Books

Below you'll find some of my other popular books that are popular on Amazon and Kindle as well. Simply click on the links below to check them out. I greatly appreciate it!

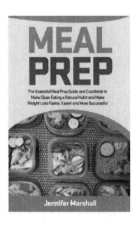

https://www.amazon.com/dp/B072TV18XF

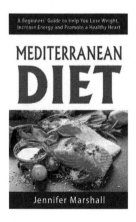

https://www.amazon.com/dp/B01M61E7H5

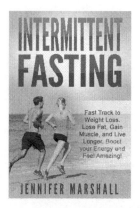

https://www.amazon.com/dp/B0154FAX34

If the links do not work, for whatever reason, you can simply search for these titles on the Amazon website to find them.

Keep Growing. And Loving.